Nature's Remedy

THIS BOOK BELONGS TO

Nature's Remedy

===============================

Green Smoothies for Fighting Cancer

AS Publishing

PUBLISHING

Published by **AS Publishing**

Follow Us to Stay Updated on New Releases

We offer our eBooks for free during the initial launch period. By following us, you will be among the first to know when a new eBook is released and have the opportunity to download it completely free of charge.

Don't miss out on our latest releases! Simply click on the link below, follow us, and stay up-to-date on all of our new eBooks.

amazon.com/author/as-publishing

Attribution: The resources utilized to design this cover were obtained from freepik.com.

Disclaimer

This book's instructions, recommendations, or methods are not intended to replace professional medical guidance, diagnosis, or care. The information in this book is only meant to be used for educational purposes; it should not be used as a replacement for professional medical advice from a healthcare provider.

The authors and publisher of this book disclaim any responsibility for any negative effects or outcomes attributable to the use of the knowledge, suggestions, or methods offered in this book. Readers should speak with their doctor before beginning any new health or wellness program.

Despite the fact that the knowledge and research upon which the information in this book is based is up-to-date, medical procedures and recommendations may alter over time.

It is advised that readers seek out additional information and keep current with healthcare trends.

The authors' views are the only ones that are expressed in this book; they do not necessarily represent the publisher's views. The authors and publisher do not endorse or recommend any companies, items, or services that are mentioned in this book.

Despite making every effort to ensure the accuracy and comprehensiveness of the information in this book, the authors and publisher make no promises or representations of any kind, either explicitly or implicitly, regarding the information's suitability, reliability, or availability.

Any risks associated with relying on the information in this book are assumed by the reader.

ISBN: 9798856082868

Contents

➢ Understanding the Role of Nutrition in Cancer Treatment and Recovery

Proper nutrition plays a crucial role in cancer treatment and recovery. Cancer and its treatments can take a toll on the body, leading to weight loss, muscle wasting, nutrient deficiencies, and a weakened immune system. Therefore, maintaining a well-balanced diet that meets the nutritional needs of cancer patients is essential to support overall health, enhance treatment outcomes, manage side effects, and promote recovery.

1. **Meeting Nutritional Needs:** Cancer patients have increased nutritional requirements due to the metabolic demands of the disease and its treatments. Adequate intake of macronutrients (carbohydrates, proteins, and fats) and micronutrients (vitamins and minerals) is necessary to provide energy, support tissue repair, and maintain optimal functioning of the body.

2. **Energy and Protein:** Cancer treatments, such as chemotherapy and radiation therapy, can increase energy expenditure and lead to weight loss. Consuming enough calories and protein is vital to prevent malnutrition, promote weight maintenance or gain, and support tissue healing. High-protein foods like lean meats, poultry, fish, eggs, legumes, and dairy products are recommended.

3. **Fruits and Vegetables:** A diet rich in fruits and vegetables provides essential vitamins, minerals,

antioxidants, and fiber. These nutrients support immune function, help fight oxidative stress caused by cancer treatments, and promote overall health. Incorporating a variety of colorful fruits and vegetables into meals and snacks is beneficial.

4. **Whole Grains:** Choosing whole grains over refined grains is recommended as they contain more fiber, vitamins, and minerals. Whole grains like whole wheat, brown rice, oats, quinoa, and barley provide sustained energy and aid in digestion.

5. **Healthy Fats:** Including healthy fats in the diet is important for cancer patients. Foods rich in omega-3 fatty acids, such as fatty fish (salmon, sardines), flaxseeds, chia seeds, and walnuts, can have anti-inflammatory effects and support heart health. Avocados, nuts, and olive oil are also good sources of healthy fats.

6. **Hydration:** Staying well-hydrated is essential for cancer patients to support overall health and prevent dehydration, which can exacerbate side effects like fatigue and nausea. Drinking an adequate amount of water and consuming hydrating foods like soups, fruits, and vegetables is recommended.

7. **Managing Side Effects:** Cancer treatments often come with side effects that can affect appetite, taste, and digestion. Working with a registered dietitian can help tailor a diet plan to manage these side effects. For instance, eating small, frequent meals, opting for bland or cold foods during

periods of nausea, and using spices or marinades to enhance flavor can be helpful strategies.

8. **Individualized Approach:** Each cancer patient is unique, and nutritional needs may vary based on the type of cancer, treatment regimen, stage of the disease, and overall health status. Therefore, it is crucial to work with a healthcare team, including registered dietitians, who can provide personalized dietary recommendations and monitor nutritional status throughout the treatment and recovery process.

In conclusion, nutrition plays a vital role in cancer treatment and recovery. A well-balanced diet that meets individual nutritional needs can help support overall health, manage treatment side effects, and enhance the body's ability to heal and recover. Working with healthcare professionals and incorporating healthy food choices can contribute to better outcomes and improve the quality of life for cancer patients.

➢ The Benefits of Green Smoothies for Cancer Patients

Green smoothies, which are packed with vitamins, minerals, and healthy leafy greens, have several benefits for cancer patients. A cancer patient's diet may benefit from including these vibrant beverages, offering a quick and delectable way to increase nutritional intake and support general health throughout treatment and recovery. Here are some key benefits of incorporating green smoothies into the diet:

1. **Nutrient-Rich:** For green smoothies, a base of leafy greens like spinach, kale, or Swiss chard is usually used. These vegetables are a great source of anti-oxidants, vital nutrients, and minerals that can boost the immune system, reduce oxidative stress, and generally improve health. They also have fiber, which promotes regular bowel movements and helps with digestion.

2. **Hydration:** Staying hydrated is crucial for cancer patients, as treatments like chemotherapy can cause dehydration. Green smoothies, often made with water or hydrating liquids like coconut water or almond milk, contribute to overall hydration. Additionally, incorporating fruits with high water content, such as melons or citrus fruits, can further enhance hydration levels.

3. **Antioxidant Support:** Cancer treatments can generate free radicals in the body, leading to oxidative stress. Green smoothies, particularly those containing leafy greens and vibrant fruits like berries or citrus, are packed with antioxidants. These antioxidants support cellular health, combat free radicals, and lower inflammation.

4. **Fiber and Digestive Health:** Maintaining a healthy digestive system is important for cancer patients, as treatments can sometimes lead to gastrointestinal side effects. Green smoothies, especially when blended with whole fruits and

vegetables, provide a good amount of dietary fiber. Fiber supports digestive health, aids in proper bowel movements, and can alleviate issues such as constipation.

5. **Energy and Weight Management:** Cancer and its treatments can cause fatigue and weight loss. Green smoothies can be a convenient way to incorporate nutrient-dense calories into the diet, providing energy and supporting weight maintenance or gain. Adding healthy fats like avocados or nut butters can further enhance the calorie content and satiety of the smoothie.

6. **Easy Nutrient Absorption:** Some cancer treatments can affect the ability of the body to absorb nutrients properly. The cellular structure of the ingredients is broken down by blending fruits and vegetables into a smoothie, making it simpler for the body to absorb the nutrients. This can help guarantee that cancer patients are getting the most benefit possible from their diet.

7. **Variety and Taste:** Green smoothies offer a wide range of flavor combinations and customization options. Cancer patients who may experience changes in taste or appetite can benefit from the versatility of green smoothies. Adjusting the ingredients to suit personal preferences can help make the smoothies more enjoyable and appealing.

It is important for cancer patients to consult with their healthcare team, including registered dietitians or nutritionists, to ensure that green smoothies fit into their individualized treatment plan. Additionally, it is advisable to choose organic produce, wash the ingredients thoroughly, and follow safe food handling practices to minimize any potential risks. During cancer treatment and recovery, incorporating green smoothies into a balanced diet can be a nourishing and revitalizing way to support general health and well-being.

➢ Exploring the Essential Nutrients Needed during Cancer Treatment

Someone who is undergoing cancer treatment needs proper nutrition in order to keep up their overall health and well-being. The objective is to give the body the necessary nutrients to support the immune system, promote healing, maintain strength, and control side effects of treatment. Here are some necessary nutrients that are frequently significant during cancer treatment, though individual nutrient needs may vary.

1. **Protein:** Protein is crucial for tissue repair, wound healing, and the production of enzymes and antibodies. Cancer treatment can increase the body's protein needs, especially if experiencing weight loss or muscle wasting.

2. **Calories and Energy:** Maintaining adequate calorie intake is essential to provide energy for the body's functions and support weight maintenance or regain. Cancer and its treatments can often lead to

decreased appetite or increased energy needs. Nutrient-dense foods like whole grains, lean proteins, healthy fats, fruits, and vegetables can help satisfy calorie requirements while supplying essential nutrients.

3. **Healthy Fats:** The creation of hormones, appropriate brain function, and the absorption of fat-soluble vitamins all depend on healthy fats, such as monounsaturated fats and omega-3 fatty acids. Avocados, almonds, seeds, olive oil, and fatty seafood like salmon or sardines are all sources of healthy fats. These fats may help the diet supply essential nutrients and promote general health.

4. **Vitamins and Minerals:** To support immune function, cellular repair, and general wellbeing during cancer treatment, it's crucial to ensure adequate intake of vitamins and minerals. Some key vitamins and minerals include:

- **Vitamin D:** Supports bone health, immune function, and overall well-being. Sunlight exposure, fortified foods, and supplementation can help meet vitamin D needs.

- **B vitamins:** Essential for energy production, nerve function, and red blood cell production. Sources include whole grains, leafy greens, legumes, and lean proteins.

- **Zinc:** Important for immune function and wound healing. Good sources include seafood, lean meats, legumes, and whole grains.

- **Iron:** Supports the production of red blood cells and energy levels. Red meat, fish, and legumes are examples of foods high in iron.

- **Magnesium:** Plays a role in muscle and nerve function, bone health, and energy production. Sources include nuts, seeds, whole grains, and leafy greens.

5. **Hydration:** Staying properly hydrated is essential during cancer treatment, as certain treatments can cause dehydration. Drinking adequate fluids, such as water, herbal teas, and clear soups, can help maintain hydration levels. Monitoring urine color and consulting healthcare professionals for individual fluid recommendations is important.

6. **Fiber:** Adequate fiber intake is important for digestive health, preventing constipation, and supporting bowel regularity. Whole grains, fruits, vegetables, legumes, and nuts are excellent sources of fiber. However, individual tolerance may vary, and it is important to manage fiber intake based on specific treatment side effects or recommendations.

Working closely with registered dietitians or nutritionists on their individualized nutrition plans based on their unique needs, treatment regimens, and any dietary restrictions is essential for people receiving cancer treatment. These professionals can provide personalized guidance on nutrient intake, meal planning, and managing treatment-related side effects to support overall health and well-being during cancer treatment.

➢ Addressing Specific Nutritional Needs for Different Types of Cancer

Cancer is a complex disease with various types, and each type may have specific nutritional considerations. While individual needs may vary, here are some general guidelines for addressing specific nutritional needs for different types of cancer:

1. **Breast Cancer:**

- **Adequate protein intake:** Protein is important for wound healing and tissue repair. Include lean sources of protein such as poultry, fish, legumes, and dairy products.

- **Phytoestrogen-rich foods:** Phytoestrogens, found in soy products, flaxseeds, and legumes, may have a protective effect against breast cancer recurrence.

- **Calcium and vitamin D:** These nutrients support bone health and are important for individuals undergoing hormone-related breast cancer treatments.

2. **Colorectal Cancer:**

- **High-fiber diet:** A diet rich in fiber from whole grains, fruits, vegetables, and legumes can support bowel regularity and help reduce the risk of recurrence.

- **Omega-3 fatty acids:** Found in fatty fish, walnuts, and flaxseeds, omega-3 fatty acids may have anti-inflammatory effects and benefit individuals with colorectal cancer.

- **Limit processed meats:** Processed meats, such as bacon and sausage, have been linked to an increased risk of colorectal cancer. Opt for lean protein sources like fish, poultry, and plant-based alternatives.

3. **Lung Cancer:**

- **Antioxidant-rich foods:** Fruits and vegetables rich in antioxidants, such as berries, leafy greens, and citrus fruits, may help protect against oxidative damage and support overall lung health.

- **Beta-carotene:** Foods high in beta-carotene, like spinach, carrots, and sweet potatoes, may be able to prevent lung cancer.

- **Avoid or limit tobacco and alcohol:** Smoking and excessive alcohol consumption are risk factors for lung cancer. It is important to avoid tobacco and limit alcohol intake.

4. **Prostate Cancer:**

- **Lycopene-rich foods:** Lycopene, found in tomatoes, watermelon, and pink grapefruit, has been associated with a lower risk of prostate cancer. Cooked tomato products, such as tomato sauce or paste, may provide more bioavailable lycopene.

- **Cruciferous vegetables:** Vegetables like broccoli, cauliflower, and Brussels sprouts contain compounds that may have protective effects against prostate cancer.

- **Healthy fats:** Including sources of healthy fats, such as avocados, nuts, seeds, and fatty fish, can support overall prostate health.

5. **Pancreatic Cancer:**

- **Pancreatic enzyme supplementation:** Pancreatic cancer can impair the production of digestive enzymes, leading to difficulties in digesting fats. Pancreatic enzyme supplementation may be necessary to aid digestion and nutrient absorption.

- **Small, frequent meals:** Eating smaller, more frequent meals throughout the day may help manage digestive symptoms and support adequate calorie intake.

- **Focus on nutrient-dense foods:** Opt for nutrient-dense foods to ensure sufficient intake of essential vitamins, minerals, and antioxidants.

Nutritional needs can vary based on the stage of cancer, treatment protocols, and individual factors. Consulting with a registered dietitian who specializes in oncology nutrition can provide personalized guidance tailored to specific needs and treatment plans. They can help develop an individualized nutrition plan and address any concerns or challenges related to diet and nutrition during cancer treatment.

➢ Green Smoothies for Cancer Patients

❖ Healing Greens Smoothie

Ingredients:

- 1 cup spinach
- 1 cup kale
- 1 medium cucumber
- 1 green apple
- 1/2 avocado
- 1/2 lemon (juiced)
- 1 cup coconut water

Instructions:

1. Wash all the greens thoroughly.
2. Peel the cucumber and chop it into chunks.
3. Core the green apple and cut it into slices.
4. Add all the ingredients to a blender.
5. Blend until you achieve a smooth consistency.
6. Serve and enjoy!

❖ Immune-Boosting Green Smoothie

Ingredients:

- 1 cup spinach
- 1 cup Swiss chard
- 1 kiwi (peeled and sliced)
- 1/2 cup pineapple chunks
- 1/2 cup green grapes
- 1/2 cup almond milk
- 1 tablespoon chia seeds

Instructions:

1. Clean the spinach and Swiss chard leaves properly.
2. Peel the kiwi and slice it into small pieces.
3. Combine all the ingredients in a blender.
4. Blend until the mixture becomes smooth and creamy.
5. Pour into a glass and sprinkle chia seeds on top.
6. Stir well and enjoy the immune-boosting green smoothie.

❖ Anti-Inflammatory Green Smoothie

Ingredients:

- 1 cup kale
- 1 cup cucumber
- 1/2 cup pineapple chunks
- 1/2 cup mango chunks
- 1/2 inch fresh ginger (peeled)
- 1 cup coconut water
- 1 tablespoon flaxseed powder

Instructions:

1. Rinse the kale and cucumber thoroughly.
2. Peel the cucumber and chop it into small pieces.
3. Cut the pineapple and mango into chunks.
4. Add all the ingredients to a blender.
5. Blend until the mixture is smooth and creamy.
6. Pour into a glass and sprinkle flaxseed powder on top.
7. Stir well and enjoy the anti-inflammatory green smoothie.

❖ Revitalizing Green Smoothie

Ingredients:

- 1 cup baby spinach
- 1 cup kale
- 1 ripe banana
- 1/2 cup green grapes
- 1/4 cup fresh mint leaves
- 1/2 cup almond milk (or any non-dairy milk)
- 1 tablespoon honey (optional)

Instructions:

1. Wash the spinach and kale leaves thoroughly.
2. Peel the banana and slice it.
3. Combine all the ingredients in a blender.
4. Blend until the mixture is smooth and creamy.
5. If desired, add honey for sweetness and blend again.
6. Pour into a glass and garnish with a sprig of fresh mint.
7. Sip and enjoy the revitalizing green smoothie.

❖ **Energizing Green Smoothie**

Ingredients:

- 1 cup spinach
- 1 cup Swiss chard
- 1 small green apple
- 1/2 cup cucumber
- 1/2 cup pineapple chunks
- 1 tablespoon fresh lime juice
- 1/2 cup coconut water
- 1 teaspoon spirulina powder (optional)

Instructions:

1. Clean the spinach and Swiss chard leaves properly.
2. Core the green apple and cut it into slices.
3. Peel the cucumber and chop it into chunks.
4. Combine all the ingredients in a blender.
5. Blend until the mixture is smooth and creamy.
6. If desired, add spirulina powder for an extra boost of nutrients and blend again.
7. Pour into a glass and serve the energizing green smoothie.

❖ Berry Green Bliss Smoothie

Ingredients:

- 1 cup spinach
- 1 cup mixed berries (such as strawberries, blueberries, and raspberries)
- 1/2 cup plain Greek yogurt
- 1/2 cup almond milk (or any non-dairy milk)
- 1 tablespoon almond butter
- 1 teaspoon honey (optional)
- Ice cubes (optional)

Instructions:

1. Wash the spinach and berries thoroughly.
2. Combine all the ingredients in a blender.
3. Blend until the mixture is smooth and creamy.
4. If desired, add a drizzle of honey for sweetness and blend again.
5. If you prefer a colder smoothie, add a few ice cubes and blend until smooth.
6. Pour into a glass and savor the berry green bliss smoothie.

❖ Creamy Avocado Spinach Smoothie

Ingredients:

- 1 cup spinach
- 1/2 avocado
- 1 small ripe banana
- 1/2 cup unsweetened coconut milk (or any non-dairy milk)
- 1 tablespoon honey or maple syrup (optional)
- 1/2 teaspoon vanilla extract

Instructions:

1. Wash the spinach thoroughly.
2. Scoop out the avocado flesh and discard the pit.
3. Peel the banana and slice it.
4. Combine all the ingredients in a blender.
5. Blend until the mixture is creamy and well combined.
6. If desired, add honey or maple syrup for sweetness and blend again.
7. Pour into a glass and indulge in the creamy avocado spinach smoothie.

❖ Tropical Green Paradise Smoothie

Ingredients:

- 1 cup spinach
- 1/2 cup chopped pineapple
- 1/2 cup chopped mango
- 1/2 cup sliced cucumber
- 1/4 cup coconut milk
- 1/4 cup orange juice
- 1 tablespoon lime juice
- A handful of ice cubes

Instructions:

1. Wash the spinach thoroughly.
2. Peel and chop the pineapple, mango, and cucumber.
3. Combine all the ingredients in a blender.
4. Blend until the mixture is smooth and creamy.
5. Add ice cubes and blend again until desired consistency.
6. Pour into a glass and enjoy the tropical green paradise smoothie.

❖ Zesty Green Citrus Smoothie

Ingredients:

- 1 cup spinach
- 1/2 cup kale
- 1 medium orange (peeled and segmented)
- 1 small lemon (juiced)
- 1/2 cup unsweetened almond milk
- 1 tablespoon honey (optional)
- A pinch of grated ginger (optional)

Instructions:

1. Clean the spinach and kale leaves properly.
2. Peel and segment the orange.
3. Juice the lemon.
4. Combine all the ingredients in a blender.
5. Blend until the mixture is smooth and well combined.
6. If desired, add honey for sweetness and grated ginger for extra zing, then blend again.
7. Pour into a glass and savor the zesty green citrus smoothie.

❖ Creamy Matcha Green Smoothie

Ingredients:

- 1 cup spinach
- 1 teaspoon matcha powder
- 1 ripe banana
- 1/2 cup unsweetened almond milk
- 1/4 cup Greek yogurt
- 1 tablespoon honey (optional)
- Ice cubes (optional)

Instructions:

1. Wash the spinach thoroughly.
2. In a blender, combine spinach, matcha powder, banana, almond milk, Greek yogurt, and honey.
3. Blend until all the ingredients are smooth and well combined.
4. If desired, add ice cubes for a chilled smoothie and blend again until smooth.
5. Pour into a glass and enjoy the creamy matcha green smoothie.

❖ Minty Watermelon Green Smoothie

Ingredients:

- 1 cup spinach
- 1 cup chopped watermelon
- 1/2 cup cucumber
- 1/4 cup fresh mint leaves
- 1/2 cup coconut water
- 1 tablespoon lime juice
- A handful of ice cubes

Instructions:

1. Wash the spinach thoroughly.
2. Remove the rind and seeds from the watermelon, and chop it into chunks.
3. Peel the cucumber and chop it into small pieces.
4. In a blender, combine spinach, watermelon, cucumber, mint leaves, coconut water, lime juice, and ice cubes.
5. Blend until all the ingredients are well combined and the mixture is smooth.
6. Pour into a glass and enjoy the refreshing minty watermelon green smoothie.

❖ Protein-Packed Green Smoothie

Ingredients:

- 1 cup spinach

- 1/2 cup kale

- 1/2 cup Greek yogurt

- 1/2 cup almond milk (or any non-dairy milk)

- 1/4 cup rolled oats

- 1 tablespoon almond butter

- 1 tablespoon chia seeds

- 1 teaspoon honey (optional)

- Ice cubes (optional)

Instructions:

1. Wash the spinach and kale leaves thoroughly.

2. In a blender, combine spinach, kale, Greek yogurt, almond milk, rolled oats, almond butter, chia seeds, and honey.

3. Blend until all the ingredients are well combined and the mixture is smooth.

4. If desired, add ice cubes for a chilled smoothie and blend again until smooth.

5. Pour into a glass and enjoy the protein-packed green smoothie.

❖ Ginger Turmeric Green Smoothie

Ingredients:

- 1 cup spinach

- 1 small banana

- 1/2 cup chopped pineapple

- 1/2 inch fresh ginger (peeled)

- 1/2 teaspoon ground turmeric

- 1 cup coconut water

- 1 tablespoon flaxseed powder

- Ice cubes (optional)

Instructions:

1. Wash the spinach thoroughly.

2. In a blender, combine spinach, banana, pineapple, ginger, turmeric, coconut water, and flaxseed powder.

3. Blend until all the ingredients are well combined and the mixture is smooth.

4. If desired, add ice cubes for a chilled smoothie and blend again until smooth.

5. Pour into a glass and savor the ginger turmeric green smoothie.

❖ Creamy Coconut Kale Smoothie

Ingredients:

- 1 cup kale
- 1/2 cup coconut milk
- 1/2 cup pineapple chunks
- 1 ripe banana
- 1 tablespoon shredded coconut
- 1 tablespoon honey (optional)
- Ice cubes (optional)

Instructions:

1. Wash the kale leaves thoroughly.
2. In a blender, combine kale, coconut milk, pineapple chunks, banana, shredded coconut, and honey.
3. Blend until all the ingredients are well combined and the mixture is smooth.
4. If desired, add ice cubes for a chilled smoothie and blend again until smooth.

5. Pour into a glass and enjoy the creamy coconut kale smoothie.

❖ Refreshing Green Cucumber Smoothie

Ingredients:

- 1 cup spinach
- 1/2 cucumber
- 1 green apple
- 1/2 cup fresh mint leaves
- 1 tablespoon lemon juice
- 1 cup coconut water
- Ice cubes (optional)

Instructions:

1. Wash the spinach thoroughly.
2. Peel the cucumber and chop it into chunks.
3. Core the green apple and cut it into slices.
4. In a blender, combine spinach, cucumber, green apple, mint leaves, lemon juice, and coconut water.
5. Blend until all the ingredients are well combined and the mixture is smooth.

6. If desired, add ice cubes for a chilled smoothie and blend again until smooth.

7. Pour into a glass and savor the refreshing green cucumber smoothie.

❖ Blueberry Spinach Power Smoothie

Ingredients:

- 1 cup spinach
- 1/2 cup blueberries
- 1/2 ripe avocado
- 1/2 cup unsweetened almond milk
- 1 tablespoon almond butter
- 1 tablespoon flaxseed meal
- 1 teaspoon honey (optional)
- Ice cubes (optional)

Instructions:

1. Wash the spinach thoroughly.

2. In a blender, combine spinach, blueberries, avocado, almond milk, almond butter, flaxseed meal, and honey.

3. Blend until all the ingredients are well combined and the mixture is smooth.

4. If desired, add ice cubes for a chilled smoothie and blend again until smooth.

5. Pour into a glass and enjoy the blueberry spinach power smoothie.

❖ Papaya Green Goddess Smoothie

Ingredients:

- 1 cup spinach
- 1 cup chopped papaya
- 1/2 cup sliced banana
- 1/4 cup Greek yogurt
- 1/4 cup coconut water
- 1 tablespoon lime juice
- 1 teaspoon honey (optional)
- Ice cubes (optional)

Instructions:

1. Wash the spinach thoroughly.

2. In a blender, combine spinach, papaya, banana, Greek yogurt, coconut water, lime juice, and honey.

3. Blend until all the ingredients are well combined and the mixture is smooth.

4. If desired, add ice cubes for a chilled smoothie and blend again until smooth.

5. Pour into a glass and savor the papaya green goddess smoothie.

❖ Creamy Spinach Mango Smoothie

Ingredients:

- 1 cup spinach
- 1 ripe mango, peeled and diced
- 1/2 cup Greek yogurt
- 1/2 cup almond milk (or any non-dairy milk)
- 1 tablespoon honey (optional)
- 1/4 teaspoon vanilla extract
- Ice cubes (optional)

Instructions:

1. Wash the spinach thoroughly.

2. In a blender, combine spinach, diced mango, Greek yogurt, almond milk, honey, and vanilla extract.

3. Blend until all the ingredients are well combined and the mixture is smooth.

4. If desired, add ice cubes for a chilled smoothie and blend again until smooth.

5. Pour into a glass and enjoy the creamy spinach mango smoothie.

❖ Kiwi Spinach Green Smoothie

Ingredients:

- 1 cup spinach
- 2 kiwis, peeled and sliced
- 1/2 cup cucumber, peeled and sliced
- 1/2 cup coconut water
- 1 tablespoon fresh lime juice
- 1 teaspoon honey (optional)
- Ice cubes (optional)

Instructions:

1. Wash the spinach thoroughly.

2. In a blender, combine spinach, sliced kiwis, sliced cucumber, coconut water, lime juice, and honey.

3. Blend until all the ingredients are well combined and the mixture is smooth.

4. If desired, add ice cubes for a chilled smoothie and blend again until smooth.

5. Pour into a glass and savor the refreshing kiwi spinach green smoothie.

❖ Pineapple Ginger Green Smoothie

Ingredients:

- 1 cup spinach
- 1 cup chopped pineapple
- 1 small banana
- 1/2 inch fresh ginger, peeled
- 1/2 cup coconut water
- 1 tablespoon lime juice
- Ice cubes (optional)

Instructions:

1. Wash the spinach thoroughly.

2. In a blender, combine spinach, chopped pineapple, banana, ginger, coconut water, and lime juice.

3. Blend until all the ingredients are well combined and the mixture is smooth.

4. If desired, add ice cubes for a chilled smoothie and blend again until smooth.

5. Pour into a glass and enjoy the refreshing pineapple ginger green smoothie.

❖ Green Apple Celery Smoothie

Ingredients:

- 1 cup spinach

- 1 green apple, cored and chopped

- 1 stalk celery, chopped

- 1/2 cup cucumber, chopped

- 1/4 cup fresh parsley leaves

- 1 cup coconut water

- 1 tablespoon lemon juice

- Ice cubes (optional)

Instructions:

1. Wash the spinach thoroughly.

2. In a blender, combine spinach, green apple, celery, cucumber, parsley leaves, coconut water, and lemon juice.

3. Blend until all the ingredients are well combined and the mixture is smooth.

4. If desired, add ice cubes for a chilled smoothie and blend again until smooth.

5. Pour into a glass and savor the green apple celery smoothie.

❖ Berry Blast Green Smoothie

Ingredients:

- 1 cup spinach
- 1/2 cup mixed berries (such as strawberries, blueberries, and raspberries)
- 1 small banana
- 1/2 cup unsweetened almond milk
- 1 tablespoon chia seeds
- 1 teaspoon honey (optional)
- Ice cubes (optional)

Instructions:

1. Wash the spinach thoroughly.

2. In a blender, combine spinach, mixed berries, banana, almond milk, chia seeds, and honey.

3. Blend until all the ingredients are well combined and the mixture is smooth.

4. If desired, add ice cubes for a chilled smoothie and blend again until smooth.

5. Pour into a glass and enjoy the refreshing berry blast green smoothie.

❖ Coconut Kale Pineapple Smoothie

Ingredients:

- 1 cup kale

- 1/2 cup chopped pineapple

- 1/2 cup coconut milk

- 1 small banana

- 1 tablespoon shredded coconut

- 1 teaspoon honey (optional)

- Ice cubes (optional)

Instructions:

1. Wash the kale thoroughly.

2. In a blender, combine kale, chopped pineapple, coconut milk, banana, shredded coconut, and honey.

3. Blend until all the ingredients are well combined and the mixture is smooth.

4. If desired, add ice cubes for a chilled smoothie and blend again until smooth.

5. Pour into a glass and savor the coconut kale pineapple smoothie.

❖ Citrus Spinach Green Smoothie

Ingredients:

- 1 cup spinach

- 1 orange, peeled and segmented

- 1/2 cup pineapple chunks

- 1 small banana

- 1/2 cup coconut water

- 1 tablespoon fresh lime juice

- 1 teaspoon honey (optional)

- Ice cubes (optional)

Instructions:

1. Wash the spinach thoroughly.

2. In a blender, combine spinach, orange segments, pineapple chunks, banana, coconut water, lime juice, and honey.

3. Blend until all the ingredients are well combined and the mixture is smooth.

4. If desired, add ice cubes for a chilled smoothie and blend again until smooth.

5. Pour into a glass and enjoy the citrus spinach green smoothie.

❖ Almond Butter Spinach Smoothie

Ingredients:

- 1 cup spinach

- 1 tablespoon almond butter

- 1 small banana

- 1/2 cup almond milk (or any non-dairy milk)

- 1 tablespoon honey (optional)

- 1/4 teaspoon cinnamon

- Ice cubes (optional)

Instructions:

1. Wash the spinach thoroughly.

2. In a blender, combine spinach, almond butter, banana, almond milk, honey, and cinnamon.

3. Blend until all the ingredients are well combined and the mixture is smooth.

4. If desired, add ice cubes for a chilled smoothie and blend again until smooth.

5. Pour into a glass and savor the almond butter spinach smoothie.

❖ Mango Avocado Green Smoothie

Ingredients:

- 1 cup spinach

- 1 ripe mango, peeled and diced

- 1/2 ripe avocado

- 1/2 cup coconut water

- 1 tablespoon lime juice

- 1 teaspoon honey (optional)

- Ice cubes (optional)

Instructions:

1. Wash the spinach thoroughly.

2. In a blender, combine spinach, diced mango, avocado, coconut water, lime juice, and honey.

3. Blend until all the ingredients are well combined and the mixture is smooth.

4. If desired, add ice cubes for a chilled smoothie and blend again until smooth.

5. Pour into a glass and enjoy the refreshing mango avocado green smoothie.

❖ Matcha Green Tea Smoothie

Ingredients:

- 1 cup spinach
- 1 teaspoon matcha green tea powder
- 1 small banana
- 1/2 cup unsweetened almond milk
- 1 tablespoon honey (optional)
- Ice cubes (optional)

Instructions:

1. Wash the spinach thoroughly.

2. In a blender, combine spinach, matcha green tea powder, banana, almond milk, and honey.

3. Blend until all the ingredients are well combined and the mixture is smooth.

4. If desired, add ice cubes for a chilled smoothie and blend again until smooth.

5. Pour into a glass and savor the refreshing matcha green tea smoothie.

❖ Tropical Spinach Coconut Smoothie

Ingredients:

- 1 cup spinach
- 1/2 cup chopped pineapple
- 1/2 cup chopped mango
- 1/2 cup coconut milk
- 1 small banana
- 1 tablespoon shredded coconut
- 1 teaspoon honey (optional)
- Ice cubes (optional)

Instructions:

1. Wash the spinach thoroughly.

2. In a blender, combine spinach, pineapple, mango, coconut milk, banana, shredded coconut, and honey.

3. Blend until all the ingredients are well combined and the mixture is smooth.

4. If desired, add ice cubes for a chilled smoothie and blend again until smooth.

5. Pour into a glass and enjoy the tropical spinach coconut smoothie.

❖ Green Grape Spinach Smoothie

Ingredients:

- 1 cup spinach
- 1 cup green grapes
- 1 small pear, cored and chopped
- 1/2 cup unsweetened almond milk
- 1 tablespoon chia seeds
- 1 teaspoon honey (optional)
- Ice cubes (optional)

Instructions:

1. Wash the spinach thoroughly.

2. In a blender, combine spinach, green grapes, chopped pear, almond milk, chia seeds, and honey.

3. Blend until all the ingredients are well combined and the mixture is smooth.

4. If desired, add ice cubes for a chilled smoothie and blend again until smooth.

5. Pour into a glass and savor the green grape spinach smoothie.

❖ Raspberry Spinach Delight Smoothie

Ingredients:

- 1 cup spinach
- 1/2 cup raspberries
- 1 small banana
- 1/2 cup unsweetened almond milk
- 1 tablespoon almond butter
- 1 teaspoon honey (optional)
- Ice cubes (optional)

Instructions:

1. Wash the spinach thoroughly.

2. In a blender, combine spinach, raspberries, banana, almond milk, almond butter, and honey.

3. Blend until all the ingredients are well combined and the mixture is smooth.

4. If desired, add ice cubes for a chilled smoothie and blend again until smooth.

5. Pour into a glass and enjoy the raspberry spinach delight smoothie.

❖ Cucumber Mint Green Smoothie

Ingredients:

- 1 cup spinach
- 1/2 cucumber, peeled and sliced
- 1 small apple, cored and chopped
- 1/4 cup fresh mint leaves
- 1/2 cup coconut water
- 1 tablespoon lime juice
- Ice cubes (optional)

Instructions:

1. Wash the spinach thoroughly.

2. In a blender, combine spinach, cucumber slices, chopped apple, mint leaves, coconut water, and lime juice.

3. Blend until all the ingredients are well combined and the mixture is smooth.

4. If desired, add ice cubes for a chilled smoothie and blend again until smooth.

5. Pour into a glass and savor the refreshing cucumber mint green smoothie.

❖ Blueberry Spinach Power Smoothie

Ingredients:

- 1 cup spinach

- 1/2 cup blueberries

- 1 small banana

- 1/2 cup unsweetened almond milk

- 1 tablespoon flax seeds

- 1 teaspoon honey (optional)

- Ice cubes (optional)

Instructions:

1. Wash the spinach thoroughly.

2. In a blender, combine spinach, blueberries, banana, almond milk, flax seeds, and honey.

3. Blend until all the ingredients are well combined and the mixture is smooth.

4. If desired, add ice cubes for a chilled smoothie and blend again until smooth.

5. Pour into a glass and enjoy the nutritious blueberry spinach power smoothie.

❖ Spinach Coconut Mango Smoothie

Ingredients:

- 1 cup spinach
- 1/2 cup chopped mango
- 1/4 cup shredded coconut
- 1/2 cup coconut milk
- 1 small banana
- 1 teaspoon honey (optional)
- Ice cubes (optional)

Instructions:

1. Wash the spinach thoroughly.

2. In a blender, combine spinach, chopped mango, shredded coconut, coconut milk, banana, and honey.

3. Blend until all the ingredients are well combined and the mixture is smooth.

4. If desired, add ice cubes for a chilled smoothie and blend again until smooth.

5. Pour into a glass and savor the tropical flavors of the spinach coconut mango smoothie.

❖ Kiwi Spinach Refresh Smoothie

Ingredients:

- 1 cup spinach
- 2 kiwis, peeled and sliced
- 1 small banana
- 1/2 cup unsweetened almond milk
- 1 tablespoon honey (optional)
- Ice cubes (optional)

Instructions:

1. Wash the spinach thoroughly.

2. In a blender, combine spinach, kiwis, banana, almond milk, and honey.

3. Blend until all the ingredients are well combined and the mixture is smooth.

4. If desired, add ice cubes for a chilled smoothie and blend again until smooth.

5. Pour into a glass and enjoy the refreshing kiwi spinach refresh smoothie.

❖ Papaya Ginger Green Smoothie

Ingredients:

- 1 cup spinach
- 1 cup chopped papaya
- 1 small banana
- 1/2 inch fresh ginger, peeled
- 1/2 cup coconut water
- 1 tablespoon lime juice
- Ice cubes (optional)

Instructions:

1. Wash the spinach thoroughly.

2. In a blender, combine spinach, chopped papaya, banana, ginger, coconut water, and lime juice.

3. Blend until all the ingredients are well combined and the mixture is smooth.

4. If desired, add ice cubes for a chilled smoothie and blend again until smooth.

5. Pour into a glass and savor the tropical flavors of the papaya ginger green smoothie.

❖ Peach Spinach Delight Smoothie

Ingredients:

- 1 cup spinach

- 1 ripe peach, pitted and sliced

- 1 small banana

- 1/2 cup unsweetened almond milk

- 1 tablespoon almond butter

- 1 teaspoon honey (optional)

- Ice cubes (optional)

Instructions:

1. Wash the spinach thoroughly.

2. In a blender, combine spinach, sliced peach, banana, almond milk, almond butter, and honey.

3. Blend until all the ingredients are well combined and the mixture is smooth.

4. If desired, add ice cubes for a chilled smoothie and blend again until smooth.

5. Pour into a glass and enjoy the peach spinach delight smoothie.

❖ Pineapple Spinach Mint Smoothie

Ingredients:

- 1 cup spinach
- 1 cup chopped pineapple
- 1 small banana
- 1/4 cup fresh mint leaves
- 1/2 cup coconut water
- 1 tablespoon lime juice
- Ice cubes (optional)

Instructions:

1. Wash the spinach thoroughly.

2. In a blender, combine spinach, chopped pineapple, banana, mint leaves, coconut water, and lime juice.

3. Blend until all the ingredients are well combined and the mixture is smooth.

4. If desired, add ice cubes for a chilled smoothie and blend again until smooth.

5. Pour into a glass and savor the refreshing pineapple spinach mint smoothie.

❖ Melon Spinach Zing Smoothie

Ingredients:

- 1 cup spinach
- 1 cup chopped melon (such as cantaloupe or honeydew)
- 1 small banana
- 1/2 cup coconut water
- 1 tablespoon fresh lime juice
- 1 teaspoon honey (optional)
- Ice cubes (optional)

Instructions:

1. Wash the spinach thoroughly.

2. In a blender, combine spinach, chopped melon, banana, coconut water, lime juice, and honey.

3. Blend until all the ingredients are well combined and the mixture is smooth.

4. If desired, add ice cubes for a chilled smoothie and blend again until smooth.

5. Pour into a glass and enjoy the refreshing melon spinach zing smoothie.

❖ Spinach Berry Blast Smoothie

Ingredients:

- 1 cup spinach
- 1/2 cup mixed berries (such as strawberries, blueberries, and raspberries)
- 1 small banana
- 1/2 cup unsweetened almond milk
- 1 tablespoon chia seeds
- 1 teaspoon honey (optional)
- Ice cubes (optional)

Instructions:

1. Wash the spinach thoroughly.

2. In a blender, combine spinach, mixed berries, banana, almond milk, chia seeds, and honey.

3. Blend until all the ingredients are well combined and the mixture is smooth.

4. If desired, add ice cubes for a chilled smoothie and blend again until smooth.

5. Pour into a glass and savor the nutritious spinach berry blast smoothie.

❖ Orange Spinach Sunrise Smoothie

Ingredients:

- 1 cup spinach

- 1 large orange, peeled and segmented

- 1 small banana

- 1/2 cup unsweetened almond milk

- 1 tablespoon flax seeds

- 1 teaspoon honey (optional)

- Ice cubes (optional)

Instructions:

1. Wash the spinach thoroughly.

2. In a blender, combine spinach, orange segments, banana, almond milk, flax seeds, and honey.

3. Blend until all the ingredients are well combined and the mixture is smooth.

4. If desired, add ice cubes for a chilled smoothie and blend again until smooth.

5. Pour into a glass and enjoy the refreshing orange spinach sunrise smoothie.

❖ Spinach Coconut Berry Smoothie

Ingredients:

- 1 cup spinach
- 1/2 cup mixed berries (such as strawberries, blueberries, and raspberries)
- 1/2 cup coconut milk
- 1 small banana
- 1 teaspoon honey (optional)
- Ice cubes (optional)

Instructions:

1. Wash the spinach thoroughly.

2. In a blender, combine spinach, mixed berries, coconut milk, banana, and honey.

3. Blend until all the ingredients are well combined and the mixture is smooth.

4. If desired, add ice cubes for a chilled smoothie and blend again until smooth.

5. Pour into a glass and savor the delightful spinach coconut berry smoothie.

❖ Spinach Avocado Delight Smoothie

Ingredients:

-   1 cup spinach
-   1/2 avocado, pitted and peeled
-   1 small banana
-   1/2 cup unsweetened almond milk
-   1 tablespoon almond butter
-   1 teaspoon honey (optional)
-   Ice cubes (optional)

Instructions:

1. Wash the spinach thoroughly.

2. In a blender, combine spinach, avocado, banana, almond milk, almond butter, and honey.

3. Blend until all the ingredients are well combined and the mixture is smooth.

4. If desired, add ice cubes for a chilled smoothie and blend again until smooth.

5. Pour into a glass and enjoy the creamy spinach avocado delight smoothie.

❖ Kale Pineapple Ginger Smoothie

Ingredients:

- 1 cup kale
- 1 cup chopped pineapple
- 1 small banana
- 1/2 inch fresh ginger, peeled
- 1/2 cup coconut water
- 1 tablespoon lime juice
- Ice cubes (optional)

Instructions:

1. Wash the kale thoroughly.

2. In a blender, combine kale, chopped pineapple, banana, ginger, coconut water, and lime juice.

3. Blend until all the ingredients are well combined and the mixture is smooth.

4. If desired, add ice cubes for a chilled smoothie and blend again until smooth.

5. Pour into a glass and savor the invigorating kale pineapple ginger smoothie.

❖ Spinach Mango Coconut Smoothie

Ingredients:

- 1 cup spinach
- 1 cup chopped mango
- 1/2 cup coconut milk
- 1 small banana
- 1 teaspoon honey (optional)
- Ice cubes (optional)

Instructions:

1. Wash the spinach thoroughly.

2. In a blender, combine spinach, chopped mango, coconut milk, banana, and honey.

3. Blend until all the ingredients are well combined and the mixture is smooth.

4. If desired, add ice cubes for a chilled smoothie and blend again until smooth.

5. Pour into a glass and savor the tropical flavors of the spinach mango coconut smoothie.

❖ Matcha Green Tea Smoothie

Ingredients:

- 1 cup spinach
- 1 teaspoon matcha green tea powder
- 1 small banana
- 1/2 cup unsweetened almond milk
- 1 tablespoon almond butter
- 1 teaspoon honey (optional)
- Ice cubes (optional)

Instructions:

1. Wash the spinach thoroughly.

2. In a blender, combine spinach, matcha green tea powder, banana, almond milk, almond butter, and honey.

3. Blend until all the ingredients are well combined and the mixture is smooth.

4. If desired, add ice cubes for a chilled smoothie and blend again until smooth.

5. Pour into a glass and enjoy the antioxidant-rich matcha green tea smoothie.

❖ Spinach Cherry Bliss Smoothie

Ingredients:

- 1 cup spinach
- 1 cup pitted cherries
- 1 small banana
- 1/2 cup unsweetened almond milk
- 1 tablespoon hemp seeds
- 1 teaspoon honey (optional)
- Ice cubes (optional)

Instructions:

1. Wash the spinach thoroughly.
2. In a blender, combine spinach, cherries, banana, almond milk, hemp seeds, and honey.
3. Blend until all the ingredients are well combined and the mixture is smooth.
4. If desired, add ice cubes for a chilled smoothie and blend again until smooth.

5. Pour into a glass and enjoy the delicious and nutritious spinach cherry bliss smoothie.

❖ Cucumber Mint Green Smoothie

Ingredients:

- 1 cup spinach

- 1 small cucumber, peeled and chopped

- 1/4 cup fresh mint leaves

- 1 small apple, cored and chopped

- 1/2 cup coconut water

- 1 tablespoon lime juice

- Ice cubes (optional)

Instructions:

1. Wash the spinach thoroughly.

2. In a blender, combine spinach, cucumber, mint leaves, apple, coconut water, and lime juice.

3. Blend until all the ingredients are well combined and the mixture is smooth.

4. If desired, add ice cubes for a chilled smoothie and blend again until smooth.

5. Pour into a glass and savor the refreshing cucumber mint green smoothie.

❖ Spinach Blueberry Power Smoothie

Ingredients:

- 1 cup spinach
- 1/2 cup blueberries
- 1 small banana
- 1/2 cup Greek yogurt
- 1 tablespoon chia seeds
- 1 teaspoon honey (optional)
- Ice cubes (optional)

Instructions:

1. Wash the spinach thoroughly.
2. In a blender, combine spinach, blueberries, banana, Greek yogurt, chia seeds, and honey.
3. Blend until all the ingredients are well combined and the mixture is smooth.
4. If desired, add ice cubes for a chilled smoothie and blend again until smooth.

5. Pour into a glass and enjoy the nutritious and antioxidant-packed spinach blueberry power smoothie.

❖ Kale Mango Banana Smoothie

Ingredients:

- 1 cup kale

- 1 cup chopped mango

- 1 small banana

- 1/2 cup unsweetened almond milk

- 1 tablespoon flax seeds

- 1 teaspoon honey (optional)

- Ice cubes (optional)

Instructions:

1. Wash the kale thoroughly.

2. In a blender, combine kale, chopped mango, banana, almond milk, flax seeds, and honey.

3. Blend until all the ingredients are well combined and the mixture is smooth.

4. If desired, add ice cubes for a chilled smoothie and blend again until smooth.

5. Pour into a glass and savor the delicious and nutrient-rich kale mango banana smoothie.

❖ Spinach Carrot Ginger Smoothie

Ingredients:

- 1 cup spinach
- 1 medium carrot, peeled and chopped
- 1 small apple, cored and chopped
- 1/2 inch fresh ginger, peeled
- 1/2 cup coconut water
- 1 tablespoon lemon juice
- Ice cubes (optional)

Instructions:

1. Wash the spinach thoroughly.

2. In a blender, combine spinach, chopped carrot, chopped apple, ginger, coconut water, and lemon juice.

3. Blend until all the ingredients are well combined and the mixture is smooth.

4. If desired, add ice cubes for a chilled smoothie and blend again until smooth.

5. Pour into a glass and enjoy the refreshing and nutritious spinach carrot ginger smoothie.

= THE END =

We appreciate you selecting this book! We hope your expectations were fulfilled or surpassed.

Please think about posting a review on social media if you liked our book. We value your opinion because it enables us to make improvements to our goods and services for future clients.

We want to thank you once more for your support and send our best to you.

PUBLISHING

Follow Us to Stay Updated on New Releases

We offer our eBooks for free during the initial launch period. By following us, you will be among the first to know when a new eBook is released and have the opportunity to download it completely free of charge.

Don't miss out on our latest releases! Simply click on the link below, follow us, and stay up-to-date on all of our new eBooks.

amazon.com/author/as-publishing